The Critical Need For Nutritional Supplementation And How To Do It

Specialty Targeted Adaptogen Foundational

Yes – You Do Need This Booklet

Unique Fitness

Utilizing Nature's Innate Qualities & Universal Excellence

Kyle McCormick, M.S., I.N.F.T.C. {Sportelesis. Inc.}

CONTENTS

Introduction

Health Care Or Sick Care?

We, as citizens of the United States and around the world, need to take responsibility for our own health, wellness, fitness, and performance. If the following areas of health/wellness are not <u>EMPHASIZED, ENCOURAGED</u>, and <u>IMPLEMENTED</u> by your primary health care provider, you need to ask yourself, – "Am I being provided health care or sick care?"

**Spiritual

**Nutrition (dietary intake)

**Sleep, Rest, Recovery

**Holistic Evaluations

**Nutritional Supplementation

**Exercise-Activity

**Personal Care

**Environment (outdoor)

**Environment (indoor)

**Energy Medicine

These are the areas emphasized, encouraged and implemented in the Unique Fitness Holistic Wellness Guideline Pyramid.

This booklet emphasizes one phase of the Holistic Wellness Guideline Pyramid; - Nutritional Supplementation. A book on comprehensive health, wellness, fitness and performance covering each phase of the pyramid will be published soon.

We would like to take this time to put the glory for this booklet and all aspects of Unique Fitness where it belongs, our *Lord Jesus Christ*. He has provided us all with amazing tools to stay and/or get well in body, soul, and spirit. By doing this we will be able to continue glorifying Him through the various ministries we are gifted with.

Although many may not think so, *everyone* is interested in wellness. Over the years I've seen many, many people neglect their health, thinking they're invincible, until a wellness challenge develops. They then wonder why they feel so lousy or are in a battle for their lives and begin to take the whole wellness concept seriously. Although it is never too late to implement nutrition and all aspects of the Unique Fitness Holistic Wellness Guideline Pyramid for miraculous wellness recoveries, it is far easier to prevent these problems in the first place.

An important note here is that we are grateful for the emergency medical programs and protocols we are blessed with. This is what our "health"care system was designed for, to keep us alive and stabilize us in these emergency situations. After this initial care, they have no real answers and we need to turn to the above areas for true and comprehensive health, wellness, fitness and performance.

Disclaimer

Even though proper nutritional supplementation, as well as all the areas of the Unique Fitness Holistic Wellness Guideline Pyramid, have been proven and have stood the test of time, most of these areas have not and never will be evaluated by the Food and Drug Administration (FDA). For this reason we are required to say that none of the products or services are intended to diagnose, treat, prevent or cure any health challenges. They are also not meant to replace the services of a qualified health care practitioner. Feel free to use and share this information with your personal holistic health care provider or contact us to begin your health, wellness, fitness and performance journey.

Mission

Unique Fitness is dedicated to providing you with the best holistic health, wellness, fitness and performance products, information, services and programs available through our Holistic Wellness Guideline Pyramid to maximize your opportunity to achieve your goals.

Vision

To continue to teach and educate all humanity on the value of a holistic wellness lifestyle while embracing the potential of the human body, soul, and spirit to be well through UNIQUE ways.

<u>U</u>=utilizing/<u>N</u>=nature's/<u>I</u>=innate/<u>Q</u>=qualities/&/<u>U</u>=universal/<u>E</u>=excellence.

"Behold, I will bring health and healing to my people and will let them enjoy abundant peace and prosperity"

Jeremiah 33:6

Nutrition 101

WHAT IS IT? DO WE NEED IT? HOW DO WE GET IT?

When talking about the general importance of nutrition and why it is so critical to our well being, I think it can be summed up with two very simple questions:

1. What are our physical bodies made of?
2. What runs {fuels} our physical bodies?

By definition, nutrition is the combination of processes by which the body receives and utilizes the materials (nutrients) necessary to maintain homeostasis. Homeostasis in this context is concerned with the maintenance of organ systems such as the respiratory, circulatory, endocrine, nervous, etc. in a dynamic state of equilibrium and balance. To put it simply, nutrition is the process by which a living being takes in food and uses it to live and grow. The food consumed is metabolized (broken down) into a vast array of life-enhancing nutrients such as carbohydrates, protein, fat, vitamins, minerals, phytonutrients, enzymes, glyconutrients, probiotics, amino acids, lignans, and more. By definition nutrients are substances obtained from food and used by the body to promote growth, maintenance, and/or repair of body cells, tissues, organs and systems.

With these simple definitions of nutrition and nutrients, I think it is evident that nutrition is critical to our health, wellness, fitness and performance, and we need to be concerned with how to supply our bodies with optimal amounts consistently each and every day.

Our entire physical body, including skin, blood, bones, tendons, nerves, cartilage, muscle, organs, hormones, RNA, DNA, etc. is synthesized (built) from the nutrients we supply it everyday. These same nutrients not only supply the raw materials to synthesize these elements, but, as mentioned earlier, they also keep the various systems of the body running efficiently. In addition, the energy nutrients of carbohydrates, proteins, and fats gives us the ability to perform our daily activities of work, play, or relaxation.

The effects of nutrition also extend from one generation to the next, and this is particularly evident during pregnancy. Research has demonstrated that poor nutrition of a woman during pregnancy can impair the health of not only her children, but also of her *grandchildren* even after they have become adults.

Also, the nutrition of a girl in her teens will help determine the soundness of her skeleton when she is eighty years old, and the nutrition of a boy in his teens will affect his chances of contracting heart disease decades later. Remember, 45 percent of the gain in bone mass occurs between conception and age eight, – another 45 percent from ages eight to sixteen, and the remaining 10 percent over the next decade. By our mid twenties we need to have accumulated our nutritional stores for a lifetime of strong and healthy bones.

C. Evert Koop, former surgeon general has stated that 8 out of the 10 leading causes of disease are dietary-related, and out of 2.1 million annual deaths, 1.6 million have their roots in poor nutrition.

The human body is composed of nearly 100 trillion cells, each one acting like a biological battery that generates life. Most if not all of these cells "turn over" and make new cells many times throughout our lifetime. Through our lifestyle habits and nutritional intake, *WE DO HAVE A CHOICE* whether vibrant, healthy cells or weakened and diseased cells replace our existing cells. The nutrients we feed our body on a daily basis have a major impact on this issue.

Scientific research has proven that most degenerative diseases are due to the cells in our bodies being replaced by weakened and diseased cells. This same principle applies to all ages, from infants to the elderly. So those people who say they feel good now and don't believe they need to eat and supplement properly, should keep in mind the choice they have made in terms of cellular "turnover." With proper lifestyle habits and nutrition, it is believed that *60 percent to 90 percent of all degenerative diseases can be prevented and or reversed*. As nutritional and wellness research continues, this is proving to be an absolute truth, and I believe it should be in the range of *90 percent to 100 percent.*

A good way to demonstrate this on a small scale is to cut an apple in halves. Cover one half with freshly squeezed lemon or orange juice, which has many of these protective nutrients. Leave the other half unprotected without the lemon or orange juice. The protected half will stay its natural color, while the unprotected half will turn brown with disease. *The very same process happens within our unprotected bodies.* Most "age spots" and many skin blemishes are actually this oxidation process reaching the surface of the body.

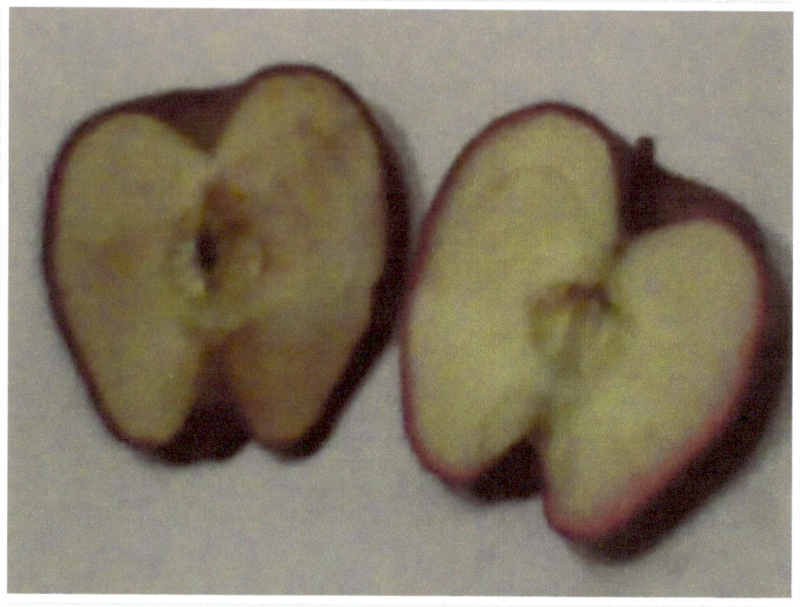

We Do Have A Choice!

Let's take a look at the various rates at which the body builds or renews healthy cells or succumbs to diseased cells, depending on what materials (nutrients) we supply our bodies.

Bone Cells = 3 ½ years

Muscle Cells = 14 months

Red Blood Cells = 4 months

Skin Cells = 1 to 2 days

Stomach Lining = 1 to 2 days

Heart Cells = 92 days

Immune Cells = 4 to 6 months

Intestinal Muscle Cells = 1 to 4 days

Organs/Glands = 3 to 6 months

Brain, Central Nervous System, and Stem Cells =
within weeks of taking glyconutrients

What do healthy cells mean to us? Healthy *cells* turn into healthy *tissues*, which turn into healthy *organs*, which turn into healthy *systems*.

Cells – Tissues – Organs – Systems = Life

We need approximately 120+ nutrients for optimal health, wellness, fitness, and performance and to build these healthy cells (16 vitamins, 8 to 12 amino acids, 3 essential fatty acids, and 92+ minerals/elements, phytonutrients, antioxidants, glycoproteins, peptides, lignans, enzymes, etc). This synergy between nutrients is very important, as even one missing nutrient can impair the effectiveness of others and lead to sub-optimal health, wellness, fitness, and performance.

An example of this synergy is the disease pellegra, which is commonly believed to be a vitamin B3 deficiency. Vitamin B3 supplementation does not always improve pellegra because, well before pellegra appears, vitamin B2, vitamin

B6, and the amino acid tryptophan are also likely to be deficient in addition to vitamin B3.

Because of this principle of synergy, these deficiencies also affect other nutrients. Vitamin B2 deficiency impairs vitamin B12 metabolism, which then impairs folic acid metabolism. Folic acid dysfunction then affects vitamin C metabolism. The resultant depletion of the body's vitamin C impairs iron absorption. Impaired iron absorption encourages excess copper absorption, which then impairs zinc metabolism, and so on.

All of these deficiency symptoms may begin as "sub-clinical deficiencies," which are marginal nutrient deficiencies not yet serious enough to cause the classic deficiency symptoms such as scurvy (vitamin C), beri beri (vitamin B1), pellegra (vitamin B3), osteoporosis (calcium), rickets (vitamin D), etc. These "sub-clinical deficiencies" will fairly quickly cause fatigue, lethargy, inability to concentrate, emotional stress and more. A prolonged "subclinical deficiency" will manifest into the classic deficiency symptoms, along with poor cellular "turnover", resulting in diseased cells, tissues, organs, and systems and causing degenerative disease.

I think we've established what nutrition is and the fact that we all need proper nutrition and nutrients to stay healthy and/or rebuild health. The question is how do we get optimal nutrition.

There are two basic ways in which we can supply these nutrients for optimal nutrition:

    1) Food intake/consumption (dietary intake)
    2) Nutritional supplementation

Dietary habits will always be an important aspect of optimal nutrition, as our diet can supply us with some nutrients, including the energy nutrients of carbohydrate, protein, and fat. In *organically* grown and raised food, there are many nutrients and nutrient compounds that are essential to our bodies functioning abilities not yet in supplement form. It's my belief we haven't even discovered many nutrients and nutrient compounds yet that will prove to be essential to our wellness. An example of this is that in one *organically* raised tomato alone, there are at least 10,000 different phytochemicals (plant chemicals) that have a variety of functions in our bodies. To date the total number of these phytochemicals that have been discovered throughout the plant kingdom is approximately 103,000.

An important point to make here is that although eating organic greatly enhances your quest for wellness by eliminating many herbicides, pesticides, and various other chemicals from your dietary intake, it does not erase the need for nutritional supplementation. This is due to a couple of issues; the product still may be harvested before peak ripeness, which reduces optimal nutrient uptake, and organic foods still begin to lose nutrient content immediately upon harvesting, so if not consumed within a few days, your nutrient intake may still be below optimal.

Look at pages 37 to 42 for a brief outline on a dietary intake program for optimal health, wellness, fitness, and performance.

<u>Supplementation: Yes or No</u>? For some reason there seems to be an ongoing debate about whether we really need nutritional supplementation to help us get these needed nutrients. I believe it has become very evident over the past several years that proper nutritional supplementation is an integral part of supplying our bodies with all the nutrients we need for optimal health, wellness, fitness, and performance. Unfortunately, I think we will see increased negative and biased media attention given to the supplement

industry. Big pharma and special interest groups would like to gain complete control over the industry, as they know quality supplements work, but as they have no patent rights on natural products, they can't gouge us with unethically increased prices and inferior products. This is another issue covered in more detail in the coming book "*Unique Way To Wellness.*" In the meantime, please use this booklet, contact us, and/or use the resources given on pages 49 to 52 for the truth about supplements.

As stated earlier, there will always be nutrients and nutrient compounds not yet discovered and therefore not in supplement form. The opposite of this is also true, there are many nutrients and nutrient compounds such as the phytochemicals, glycoproteins, enzymes, phytosterols, betalains, xanthones, etc. that are so very easily destroyed with any type of processing that the only way to get optimal amounts for our health is through proper supplementation. There are also numerous life sustaining nutrients in the discarded parts of many foods (rind, skin, bark, roots, seeds, leaves, etc.) that without being in supplement form would never lend their benefits to us.

At one time I believed in the concept of getting all the necessary nutrients through dietary intake alone. Further research and study has made me a firm believer in the absolute necessity of proper nutritional supplementation in the quest for optimal health, wellness, fitness, and performance. I am now a regular consumer of high-quality nutritionals and enjoy excellent health.

Some of what this continued research and study has revealed is as follows:

**As stated earlier, we need *120+ nutrients* for optimal health. Of these 120+ nutrients, we need 92+ minerals/ mineral elements. The soil in the United States provides at best *8 to 16* of these minerals. *Remember synergy.* The late Dr. Linus Pauling, recipient of 2 Nobel Prizes stated, "You can trace every sickness, every disease, and every ailment to a mineral deficiency." This is a very realistic statement made by Dr. Pauling as consumption of the high-quality minerals found in food and/or supplements is one of the best ways to keep the body's pH levels balanced. A highly acidic body is a major cause of nearly all sicknesses, diseases, and ailments that humans encounter.

**Refined wheat flour loses the following nutrients – (deficiency symptoms in parenthesis):

*Chromium = 98 percent {diabetes like conditions, inability to use glucose}

*Iodine = 90 percent to 100 percent (fatigue, weight gain, dry hair and skin) – Iodine is being replaced with bromine which competes with iodine for absorption.

*Vitamin E = 96 percent (dry skin, sexual dysfunction, heart disease)

*Dietary Fiber = 90 percent (high cholesterol, colon disorders, weight gain, constipation, hemorrhoids, blood sugar imbalance)

*Cobalt = 90 percent (nerve function disorder)

*Magnesium = 84 percent (weakness, confusion, muscle spasms, behavioral disturbances, depressed pancreatic hormone secretion,cardiovascular disease)

*Zinc = 78 percent (growth failure in children, sexual retardation, loss of appetite, poor wound healing)

*Vitamin B6 = 78 percent (low energy, elevated homocysteine, muscle weakness, anemia, nervous disorders, skin rash, migraines)

*Potassium = 77 percent (muscle weakness, paralysis, confusion, cardiovascular disease)

*Copper = 68 percent (anemia)

*Calcium = 60 percent {stunted growth in children, bone loss}

*Folic Acid = 50 percent (birth defects)

*Selenium = 16 percent {anemia}

In addition to these nutrients refined wheat flour also loses many additional vitamins, phytonutrients (95 percent), and trace elements. These missing nutrients in refined/processed foods are critical to immune function, cell communication, appetite control, preventing free radical damage, fetal brain development, and many additional functions. Attempting to enhance these processed/refined foods comes up woefully short in terms of balanced nutrition. Most refined products are "enriched" with only some B vitamins, vitamin D, calcium, and iron salts after more than 20 natural nutrients have been removed during processing. The "enriched" nutrients are usually of inferior quality, resulting in poor bioavailability for humans.

These nutrient losses are true of all highly processed and refined foods.

**In 1940 wheat provided 40 percent protein – Today it provides less than 9 percent

**Freezing meats destroys 50 percent of vitamins B1 and B2 – and 70 percent of pantothentic acid.

**Processing meats destroys 50 percent to 70 percent of vitamin B6 (which can result in muscle weakness, anemia, nervous disorders, skin rashes, kidney stones, and convulsions).

**A tree ripened organic orange has 180 mg of vitamin C. Many store bought oranges have little to no vitamin C.

**U.S. Senate Document #264 of the 74th congress session stated, *"Soils are mineral deficient. The only way to get sufficient mineral intake is through mineral supplementation."* This was written in 1936.

**In 1994 congress unanimously passed the Dietary Supplement Health and Education Act (DSHEA), stating that there is a *definite link between taking dietary supplements and disease prevention.*

**In 1948, one cup of spinach provided 24 mcg of iron. Today one cup of spinach provides 2 mcg of iron (inability to concentrate, pallor headaches, and weakness).

**Meat from grass-fed animals has half the saturated fat of that from grain-fed animals

**Chickens that feed on pasture have 21 percent less total fat, 30 percent less saturated fat, 28 percent fewer calories, and 100 percent more omega 3 fatty acids (healthy fat)} than chickens given high-energy specialty feed. The eggs of the pasture-raised chickens also have 400 percent more omega 3 fats.

**Between 1963 and 2000 the vitamin C in spinach dropped by 45 percent

**In October of 2002 the *Journal of the American Medical Association* stated – "that research has proven that every adult should take a multi vitamin since it is impossible to obtain all the necessary nutrients from our daily food intake today."

This is only a very small list of nutrient depletion in today's food supply.

It is also estimated that we are exposed to *1000 times* more toxins in *one day* than our grandparents were exposed to in a *lifetime*. {heavy metals, pesticides, herbicides, radiation, carbon monoxide, etc}. This further enhances our need for high-quality nutrients in our daily regime.

Other reasons to use high quality supplementation include:

> poor digestion, hot coffee/tea/spices, alcohol, smoking, laxatives, fad diets, over cooking, food processing, convenience foods, antibiotics, food allergies, crop nutrient losses, soil depletion, accidents, illness, stress, pms, teenagers, pregnancy, oral contraceptives, light eaters, elderly, lack of sunlight, poor bioavailability, low body reserves, athletes/highly active, food storage, food shipping, shelf life, pesticides, herbicides, etc.

> The common thread extending from this list is that it encompasses everyone. No one can expect optimal nourishment without proper high quality supplementation.

Review the deficiency symptoms of some of these nutrients. Do you know anyone with any of these symptoms? Could it be that their only problem is a nutritional deficiency??

WE DO HAVE A CHOICE

What does all this sub-optimal nutrition mean to us?

**98 percent of the population is not getting the nutrients their bodies need on a daily basis.

**Men with the lowest amount of vitamin C have a 62 percent increased risk of cancer and due to the comprehensive wellness benefits of vitamin C a 57 percent increased risk of dying from any cause.

**80 million people have elevated cholesterol, 60 million have high blood pressure, 41 million have arthritis, and 16 million have diabetes.

**9 out of 10 people will die from heart disease or cancer, diseases virtually unknown in the early 1900's – At the turn of the century, cancer was 1 in 40 people, not 1 in 3 like today.

**Children's asthma and diabetes are up by 800 percent in recent years. Trans fatty acids play a huge role in both of these health challenges.

**People who die from heart attacks have lower heart magnesium levels than people of the same age who die from other causes.

**According to a study by Dr. R. Shulman (*British Journal of Psychiatry*), – 48 of his 59 psychotic patients had folic acid deficiencies. Studies have shown that symptoms of mental illness can be "switched off and on" by altering vitamin levels in the system.

**An essential fatty acid (EFA) deficiency in a pregnant woman's diet can impair the development of the baby's brain and retinas.

**A single nutrient deficiency can endanger the whole body. Remember synergy!

**More than 4,000 people a day have a heart attack in the United States. Selenium deficiency increases heart disease risk by 3 times.

Again, this is only a very partial list of the detrimental effects of sub-par nutrition.

What can optimal nutrition and supplementation mean to us?

**The trace mineral selenium reduces prostrate cancer by 63 percent,colorectal cancer by 58 percent, and lung cancer by 46 percent.

**Women with high levels of vitamin E reduce their breast cancer risk by up to 5 times.

**Vitamin E reduces the risk of heart attack by 75 percent.

**Children show increased intelligence and attention span with supplementation, – especially the essential fatty acids – ("*The Lancet*").

**Nine daily servings of antioxidants through food intake and/or supplementation can cut your risk of heart disease by 70 percent, - diabetes by 40 percent, - and lung cancer by 30 percent, - (studies conducted by Harvard Medical Center, UCLA Medical Center, *NewEngland Journal of Medicine*, National Cancer Institute, American Heart Association, and International Diabetes Institute).

**Consuming 1,400 mg per day of calcium can reduce the risk of cancer by 77 percent (Creighton University study).

**Regular intakes of a high-quality multi-vitamin and mineral supplement can reduce both pre and post menopausal symptoms by 70 percent (double blind study by *Journal of American College of Nutrition and Journal of Reproductive Medicine*).

**Food cravings can be eliminated or reduced. Food cravings are nature's way of letting us know we are not getting balanced nutrition in our system.

**The death rate from heart disease is 48 percent lower in those with a high intake of vitamin C.

**Zinc supplementation improves sperm count and symptoms of Alzheimer's.

Once again, this is a very partial list of optimal nutrient benefits.

NUTRITIONAL THERAPY – REDUCES RECOVERY TIME

	Enzyme/ Nutrition Group	Control Group/ No Enzymes or Supplements
Hematoma	6.62 days	15.59 days
Swelling	4.25 days	9.82 days
Movement Restriction	5.04 days	12.62 days
Inflammation	3.83 days	10.56 days
Unfit for training	4.18 days	10.23 days
Unfit for Work	2.00 days	5.29 days

FOOD IS THE ORIGINAL
MEDICINE AND REMAINS THE BEST MEDICINE!

The RDA-'s/ROI-'s Versus ODI-'s

The RDAs'/ROIs' (recommended dietary intake/recommended optimal intake) are too low for optimal health, wellness, fitness, and performance. They are general guidelines on the amount of each nutrient your body needs to function properly. It is relatively easy to exceed these minimal requirements, which will not negatively affect health, wellness, fitness, and performance and in many instances will give added benefits. The RDA-'s are basically the minimum amount of a nutrient needed to stay alive and are based on average sized, healthy adults. They are believed to be calculated with plenty of margin of safety for this population. The RDA-'s should not be confused with requirements for a specific individual and have not been set for all recognized nutrients. While these allowances are thought_to provide an adequate buffer in cases of nutritional stress, they will not supply the increased needs of someone whose reserves are depleted by pollution, disease, medications, metabolic disorders, illness, injury, nutrient losses in the growing, harvesting, processing and preparation of foods, or in a fitness or sports conditioning program. *In other words, everyone.*

If you are in search of optimal health, wellness, fitness, and performance, the RDA-'s are simply insufficient.

In addition, the human body is not a 100 percent efficient machine in terms of nutrient absorption. Depending on the nutrients involved, the absorption rate of some is only 15 percent to 30 percent of intake. So if you are only getting 100 percent of the RDA-'s, I would highly recommend better dietary habits and supplementation to cover even these minimal requirements.

ODI-'s (optimal dietary intake) are amounts of nutrients needed for vibrant, good health. The ODI-'s account for the real-life, everyday physical, mental, and/or environmental stresses we all encounter. The synergy through balanced dietary intake and proper nutritional supplementation will innately balance our nutritional needs.

HOW TO SUPPLEMENT

This brings us to the nuts and bolts in terms of how to build a nutritional supplement program. Building a supplement program can be viewed in much the same way as building a house. You don't start building a house with the roof; you begin with a solid foundation. This is exactly what needs to happen with supplementation. Get a solid foundation built, and everything else in terms of specific needs will come together much more efficiently. In nutrition, this foundation is needed because of synergy. Remember synergy? Synergy is the combined effect the of two or more agents that is greater than the effect of either of the agents used alone. (see pages 5 and 6).

START WITH THE FOUNDATION

Along with the foundation, there are three additional phases involved in building a proper nutritional supplementation program:

1) Foundational Phase

2) Adaptogen Phase

3) Targeted Phase

4) Specialty Phase

In conjunction with your dietary intake, this will allow you to meet your ODI's each and every day for optimal health, wellness, fitness, and performance.

1) FOUNDATIONAL PHASE:

Everyone needs this phase! Just like building a house, this gives your body a solid base to build upon. A good foundational product will allow the adaptogens and targeted nutritionals to perform their duties much more efficiently. Foundational products will provide a wide variety of needed vitamins, minerals, essential fatty acids, amino acids, phytonutrients, antioxidants, beneficial flora, etc. to give the body the materials to "build" healthy cells.

Cells – Tissues – Organs – Systems = Life

2) ADAPTOGEN PHASE:

Everyone also needs this phase. Adaptogens work to restore your vitality and normal functioning despite internal and external stress factors, including; physical, environmental, and emotional. Just as the foundational products allow adaptogens to function more efficiently, adaptogens in turn enhance the effectiveness of the foundationals. Adaptogens work to nourish and support the entire body or individual organs where needed to promote optimal health, wellness, fitness, and performance while innately bringing the body into homeostasis.

3) TARGETED PHASE:

Those with specific health, wellness, fitness, and/or performance challenges need to incorporate the targeted phase. Targeted nutritionals are specific formulations of vitamins, minerals, amino acids, phytonutrients, glyconutrients, essential oils, etc. that target these specific challenges. Whatever the challenge may be, there is a targeted formulation to greatly benefit it.

4) SPECIALTY PHASE:

This phase is for acute/occasional health, wellness, fitness, and/or performance issues such as illness or injury. These specialty products are usually used over a relatively short term and/or periodically until the issue is resolved. Think of the specialty phase as your holistic medicine chest.

There it is, the essence of a sound nutritional supplementation program. Begin with a solid foundation, add a high-quality adaptogen, and for those with specific health, wellness, fitness, and/or performance challenges, add a targeted formulation. For those acute/occasional issues that "pop" up, a specialty application may be warranted. By doing this you will create that all important synergistic balance.

In summary, a nutritional supplementation program is "built" around five variables: *product, dosage, times, duration,* and *purpose.* If you feel the need to alter any of these variables for maximum benefits, consult with a nutritionally oriented health care professional. Some conditions that may warrant alterations include: size, age, gender, activity level, current health status, and environment.

Nutritional Supplementation Guideline Pyramid

HOW TO BUILD A SUPPLEMENT PROGRAM

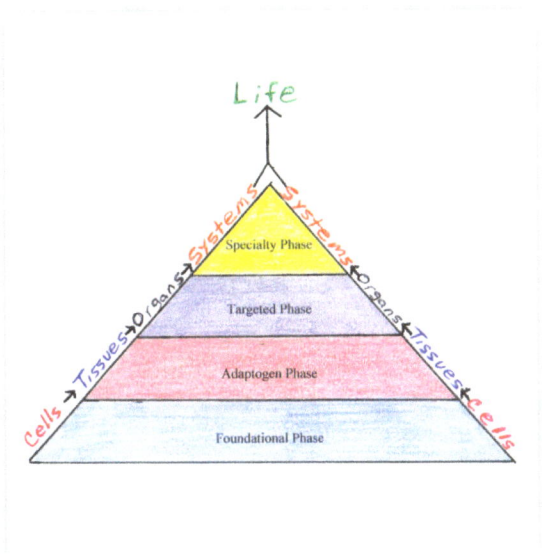

Combine this with the complete Unique Fitness Holistic Wellness Guideline Pyramid, and it will be *impossible* to not improve upon your health, wellness, fitness, and/or performance.

See page 43 for an outline of the complete pyramid.

SUPPLEMENT GUIDELINES

Name_____ Date_____

<u>Foundational:</u>

Product : Select product from the following list or web sites

Dosage : Follow product directions for all foundationals

Times : Follow product directions

Duration : Continuous, may alternate products from the following lists or company web sites located in the resources

Purpose : Solid nutritional foundation

Note : For optimal results it is best to stay on the same product for a minimum of 2 months before changing, as this will give each product time to work and balance the system.

<u>Adaptogen:</u>

Product : Select product from the following list or web sites

Dosage : Follow product directions (see note)

Times : Follow product directions (see note)

Duration : Continuous, may alternate products from the following list or company web sites located in the resources

Purpose : Nourish and support where the body needs additional benefits

Note : With most adaptogens, you can increase the dosage up to double the suggested use for added benefits. For best results increase dosage slowly and divide throughout the day. As with the foundationals, remain on the same product for a minimum of 2 months before changing.

Targeted:

Product : Select product from the following list or web sites

Dosage : Follow product directions (see note)

Times : Follow product directions (see note)

Duration : Short or long term, depending on wellness challenge – (may even be continuous) – may alternate products from the following list or company web sites located in the resources.

Purpose : Target specific health, wellness, fitness, or performance issues

Note: With most targeted products, you can again increase the dosage up to double the suggested use for added benefits. For best results increase dosage slowly and divide throughout the day. Again, remain on the same product for a minimum of 2 months before changing.

Specialty:

Product : Select product from the following list or web sites, You can also supply your holistic medicine chest with a variety of products

Dosage : Follow product directions

Times : Follow product directions

Duration : Usually short term and/or occasional until wellness issue is resolved

Purpose : Additional nutritional support and specialty wellness needs

Note : Keep your holistic medicine chest stocked with nature's medicine

On the following pages you will find several outstanding products for each phase of the nutritional supplementation guidelines. After each product is the name of the company it comes from. These are the very same companies and products we use in our nutritional supplement programs and are among the very best you will find anywhere. Each company is dedicated to staying current with emerging research and supplements and adding to the product lines as warranted.

Look on pages 49 to 52 for the company web addresses. Feel free to log on and take a look around, as there are additional products and a wealth of information that can be very beneficial to your health, wellness, fitness, and performance. You will also find additional web sites that are loaded with wellness information that you can't afford to be without.

To order and use any of these products or others found on the web sites, you can do the following:

1) Order directly from the companies.

2) Find a wellness store/clinic in your area and ask them to order the products in.

3) Contact us at Unique Fitness. We do mail order (see contact info on page 55).

You will find many, many outstanding products both in this booklet and on the web sites. Please don't get overwhelmed and confused. Keep it simple. That is exactly why we have created this Nutritional Supplement Guideline Pyramid. Fill each phase as needed, and let the health, wellness, fitness, and performance benefits begin. With the advancements in nutritional sciences and delivery systems, this is very realistic today. It is even more realistic as you incorporate additional aspects of the comprehensive Unique Fitness Holistic Wellness Guideline Pyramid (page 43).

We are 100 percent confident in each and every company mentioned and the products they offer. They will provide the wellness benefits you are seeking. If you feel the need to match the various products in each phase to your unique bio-individuality, seek out a wellness practitioner who uses muscle testing. This is a simple non-invasive technique that will provide you with the products best suited for the unique you.

You probably will find two, three or more products in each phase that work equally well. There is no problem in switching these products from time to time. As mentioned before, it is best if you stay on a set regimen for two to three months to allow the full benefits to blossom.

FOUNDATIONAL PRODUCTS

<u>High Potency Multi Vit A Min , Ultra Laboratories</u> – A gluten free and vegetarian product containing therapeutic dosages of more than 50 premium, high-potency vitamins, minerals, antioxidants, co-enzymes, carotenoids, and tocotrienols.

<u>Optimum Multi-Vitamin & Mineral Formula , Clayton Naturals</u> – A synergistically balanced supplement to produce the maximum benefit, without the mega-dose effect. Made from only the purest and most natural ingredients and free from dyes, fillers, and animal products.

<u>Platform, Lifelink</u> – One of the most potent and balanced multi vitamin and mineral supplements available. Platform contains vitamins, antioxidants, minerals (electrolyte, macro and trace), essential amino acids, brain nutrients, detoxifiers, and cancer fighters.

<u>Living Green Liquid-Gel Multi For Men , Irwin Naturals</u> – Uses powerful botanicals from whole living plants that are targeted to benefit the unique nutritional profile of men. The Living Green Liquid-Gel Multi For Men combines over 100 nutrients, vitamins, and minerals including pumpkin seed oil and saw palmetto for prostrate health.

<u>Living Green Liquid-Gel Multi For Women, Irwin Naturals</u> – Uses powerful botanicals from whole living plants that are targeted to benefit the unique nutritional profile of women. This outstanding formula combines over 100 nutrients, vitamins, and minerals including folic acid, omega 3 oils and cranberry.

<u>Kids Berry Licious Super Multi, Irwin Naturals</u> – A good tasting and chewable multi vitamin and mineral for kids with serious nutrition. Berry Licious is gluten free and naturally sweetened,

with 13 vitamins and minerals along with whole fruits and vegetables, including; broccoli, carrots, kale, and raspberries.

Whole Body Daily Multi Vitamin For Women, Irwin Naturals – Much more than an ordinary multi vitamin, this whole body daily multi vitamin addresses ten specialized areas to benefit women's health, energy, digestion, immune function, memory, and concentration. Whole Body Daily Multi Vitamin For Women includes; nutrient dense fruits, and vegetables, green super foods, amino acids, omega fatty acids, and anti-oxidant protection.

Vitality Super Greens, Body Ecology – An excellent source of complete, easily assimilated proteins, enzymes, vitamins, minerals, lignans, essential fatty acids, nucleic acids, and beneficial micro flora. This alkalizing combination will nourish the inner ecosystem while soothing and rebuilding the intestinal lining.

Tachyonized Spirulina, Tachyon – An incredibly nutrient dense food, spirulina contains every nutrient required to sustain our lives, with the exception of water. This nutrient profile includes rare essential fatty acids, carbohydrates, vitamins, minerals, phytochemicals, antioxidants, carotenoids, beta glucans, sulfolipids, protein, vitamin B12, beta carotene, chlorophyll, lutein, and zeaxanthin. This product is also tachyonized, which increases its benefits exponentially

Green Power, Starwest Botanicals – A blend of potent plant foods packed with all the vitamins, minerals, and enzymes that our bodies need to encourage optimal health and well being. Made with all organic barley grass powder, wheat grass powder, spirulina, spinach, alfalfa leaf powder, kelp powder, dulse leaf powder, orange peel powder, beet root powder, dandelion leaf powder, lemon peel powder, and ginkgo leaf powder.

Omni Jr., Davinci Laboratories – Provides older children, teens, and adults with a complete multi-vitamin containing 33 vitamins and minerals that are frequently inadequately supplied in their daily diet. Omni Jr. contains higher potencies than typical children's supplements in a combination that gives special attention to balance and bioavailability.

Multi-Vitamin Plus Daily Formula, Alacer Corp – A multi-vitamin without the pill. This is a tasty, fizzy drink that has all the vitamins and minerals you want in a multi-vitamin. Multi-Vitamin Plus comes in a great tasting cherry pomegranate flavor.

Only One Liquid-Gel Multi With Iron, Irwin Naturals – Provides comprehensive nutritional support in "only one" liquid soft-gel per day. Packed with vitamins, minerals and trace nutrients.

Men's 45+ Multi Vit-A-Min, Ultra Laboratories – A clinically proven formula for prostrate, heart, and bone support that is tailored to meet the specific health needs of men over forty-five.

Women's 45+ Multi Vit-A-Min, Ultra Laboratories – A clinically proven formula for bone, heart, and hormone support that is tailored to meet the specific health needs of women over forty-five.

ADAPTOGEN PRODUCTS

Rainforest Exotic Fruit Complex, Ultra Laboratories – A unique blend of six of the most powerful exotic fruit ingredients in the world including acai, mangosteen, pomegranate, camu camu, goji, and noni. The wellness benefits are endless.

Mangosteen, Ultra Laboraotries – A tropical fruit originating from East Asia, mangosteen is loaded with powerful antioxidants to help regulate the immune system, promote blood sugar balance, and stimulate energy production. Mangosteen contains xanthones, one of the most potent antioxidants known to man.

Goji Berry, Ultra Laboratories – A nutrient-dense fruit containing potent antioxidants, zeaxanthin, flavonoids, vitamins, minerals, and some particularly intriguing polysaccharides that are unique to goji berries. These polysaccharides (glyconutrients) provide amazing wellness benefits including inhibiting skin aging, stimulating cellular health, and increasing longevity.

Resveratrol, Ultra Laboratories – Found largely in the skins of red grapes, resveratrol will promote heart health, good circulation, and optimal liver health. As with many super foods, resveratrol is loaded with balanced nutrients to benefit many aspects of health, wellness, fitness and performance, including metabolism regulation through activating sirtuin proteins.

Coral Calcium Plus, Ultra Laboratories – An excellent product that contains a balance of calcium and magnesium, plus vitamin D3. Coral calcium also contains a number of trace minerals to enhance bone health, enzyme activity, protein synthesis, energy production, and the Ph balance of the system.

<u>MSM and Vitamin C, Ultra Laboratories</u> –
MSM (methylsulphonylmethane) is a naturally occurring sulfur compound and is the fourth most needed element next to oxygen, water, and salt in human nutrition. MSM is a major player in healthy cellular "turnover." Vitamin C enhances MSM's bioavailability, along with providing all the wellness benefits of vitamin C wound healing, nutrient absorption, bone health, skin health, blood vessel health, and more.

<u>Colostrum, Ultra Laboratories</u> – High grade "first milk" colostrum is very high in immune supporting and growth factors, – 25 percent IgG (immunoglobulin G) and elevated levels of IGF (insulin like growth factor-1) and EGF (epidermal growth factor). Works to boost the underactive immune system as well as regulate an overactive immune system. Powerful healing factors and anti-aging benefits.

<u>Ginza-Plus, Irwin Naturals</u> – Ginza Plus combines 5 powerful adaptogenic nutrients that have a balancing effect on the body during times of stress. This formula provides support in three distinct areas energy and mood, general wellness, and sexual support.

<u>Innergy Biotic, Body Ecology</u> – A probiotic energy drink that is gluten free. Innergy Biotic will boost energy, improve immunity, and prevent early aging.

<u>Essential Balance Jr., Omega Nutrition</u> – Your family will love this nutritious, great-tasting butterscotch-flavored EFA blend. It provides the ideal 2:1 omega 3 to omega 6 ratio for growing minds and bodies. Just mix with juice, yogurt, porridge, applesauce or something similar. You can help make sure your children or grandchildren get the nutrients they need.

<u>Tachyonized Siberian Ginseng (eleutherococcus), Tachyon</u> – Increases the body's resistance to environmental factors and

illness. This tonic increases the vitality and well-being of the entire body.

Tachyonized Enhancer, Tachyon – A blend of some of the world's most exotic herbs from South America, Africa, Asia and across the globe. This formula will enhance stamina, performance, and vitality. Contains kola nut, nettles, catuaba, korean ginseng, yohimbe, siberian ginseng, muira puama, saw palmetto, oat straw, epimedium, and damiana.

Essential Balance 3-6-9 Oil Blend, Omega Nutrition – This supplement is essential for daily use because our bodies depend on EFA-'s for normal functioning cells. EFA-'s are building blocks for cell membranes and produce hormone-like substances necessary for energy metabolism, cardiovascular health, and immune health.

Kenzen Ciaga, Nikken – With organic macqui-acai super fruit blend, CiagaV is one of the most potent nutritionals available. The macqui berry and acai berry have among the highest antioxidant value of any fruits, with exceptionally high levels of anthocyanins.

Royal Jelly, Beehive Botanicals – A nutrient dense product that contains all the essential amino acids plus many vitamins and minerals. Royal Jelly can enhance overall health, wellness, fitness, and performance.

TARGETED PRODUCTS

<u>Ultra Whey- 26, Unique Fitness Private Labeling</u> – An excellent protein powder to help in getting the needed protein in the diet for optimal health, wellness, fitness, and performance. Contains whey protein isolate, natural and artificial flavors, xanthan gum, stevia, and soy lecithin.

<u>Cardio Health, Ultra Laboratories</u> – A gluten-free and vegan product with therapeutic dosages of synergistic nutrients shown to support overall cardiovascular and artery health. Some of these outstanding nutrients include delta tocotrienols, (vitamin E), tumeric root extract, pomegranate, green tea, hawthorne, garlic, noni fruit, and more.

<u>Osteo Bone Health, Ultra Laboratories</u> – A gluten-free product with therapeutic dosages of essential nutrients to benefit optimal bone density and maintain "calcium favorable" pH levels. Nutrients include albion mineral chelates, potassium, vitamin K2, MSM, tumeric extract, magnesium, calcium, alfalfa, chlorella, and more.

<u>Creatine Triphase, Unique Fitness Private Labeling</u> – Creatine Triphase, which includes creatine monohydrate, creatine phosphate, and creatine pyruvate, will assist in putting on lean mass, add muscle strength, and improve performance. Creatine is essential for producing ATP (adenosine triphosphate), which is the fuel for motion involving musclecontraction. When ATP is depleted you are fatigued and lose training intensity and focus.

<u>UC-II Joint Formula, Ultra Laboratories</u> – UC-II contains undenatured collagen II, tumeric root (mervia phytosome), grape seed extract, pomegranate extract, and ginger root powder. Collagen is the protein building block in the skin, ligaments, tendons, bone, cartilage, blood vessels, and other

connective tissue. This product is clinically proven to be 200 percent more effective in promoting joint health, mobility, and flexibility than 1500mg glucosamine and 1200mg chondroitin.

NooRacetam, Lifelink – A nootropic supplement and cognitive enhancer that facilitates learning and improves memory, along with improving blood circulation. NooRacetam will make it easier to learn and remember things.

Cardiopeptase, Lifelink – An anti-inflammatory enzyme that may reduce discomfort, coughs, and hardened arteries. This "protease" enzyme can destroy fibrous proteins and clear them from the body resulting in various additional benefits for concerns such as sprains and torn ligaments, carpal tunnel, pulmonary disease, blood clots, arterial plaques, and more.

System – Six, Irwin Naturals – Powerful weight loss support with metabolism boosters and carbohydrate metabolizers. This is a complete formula that provides six support systems to assist in weight loss, exercise endurance, energy, mood, metabolism, carbohydrate support, and anti-oxidant protection.

System Six with Xenedrol, Irwin Naturals – A high-performance weight loss support system for men. This complete formula helps you support your lean, ripped physique in six ways: lean muscle support, xenedrol effect, attitude and brain chemistry, fuel, carbohydrate support, and thermogenesis.

Vision Sharp Multi-Nutrient Eye Health, Irwin Naturals – Powerful daily protection to slow the effects of age-related vision degeneration. A combination of vision specific minerals, botanicals, and powerful anti oxidants to protect and support eye tissue. Includes bilberry, citrus bioflavonoids, zeaxanthin, lutein, vitamin A, vitamin C, and more.

Emergen-C Kidz, Emergen-C – Each packet fizzes in water to provide 250 mg of vitamin C plus zinc, quercetin, and other antioxidants for immune system support, 5 B vitamins that play a key role in energy metabolism, and essential minerals and electrolytes to help active kids stay healthy.

Tachyonized General Health Tonic for Babies & Small Children, Tachyon- This compound is useful for most of the day-to-day health problems of children, specifically for feverish conditions due to colds, flu, cough, diarrhea, upset stomach, and colic.

Kenzen Joint, Nikken – An advanced formula that nutritionally supports cartilage, bone, and connective tissue repair. Contains cetyl myristoleate (CMO), myristoleic acid, myristic acid, oleic acid, palmitic acid, palmitolericacid, linoleic acid and steric acid.

Acai Meal Replacement, Ultra Laboratories – A healthy, nutritional blend of acai berry and powerful cleansing ingredients that supports a proper balance of healthy digestion and weight loss/maintenance for total overall health. Contains 25 grams of protein per serving.

COQ-10, Lifelink – COQ-10 is a very powerful fat-soluable anti-oxidant effective in maintaining optimal energy levels and preventing free radical damage. COQ-10 is critical for not only heart health but for complete cardiovascular wellness. COQ-10 can also benefit neurologic function, immune health, skin, and cancer protection.

SPECIALTY PRODUCTS

<u>Lakanto, Body Ecology</u> – An all-natural sweetener that is a zero glycemic index and non-caloric sugar substitute. Lakanto can be used just like sugar, as its sweetness is equivalent. Lakanto is great for cooking and baking, has no aftertaste, and does not cause cavities. Finally, the no calorie, healthy natural sweetener that's just like sugar.

<u>Allergy Health, Ultra Laboratories</u> – A gluten-free and vegan product with therapeutic dosages of synergistic nutrients that have been shown to improve symptoms of allergy-season challenges caused by natural pollen, air borne pollutants, dander, and other related allergens. Allergy Health contains vitamin C (non-acidic), quercetin, nettle leaf, n-acetyl cysteine, bromelain, eyebright herb, and more.

<u>Melatonin, Ultra Laboratories</u> – Helps the body in regulating the natural sleep cycle. As we age our levels of melatonin can decline. Melatonin also acts as an anti-oxidant hormone that can protect brain cells from oxidative damage.

<u>PriMeric, Lifelink</u> – Curcumin, the yellow substance in turmeric is the main ingredient in PriMeric. In India and China, curcumin has a long history of medicinal use. Recent research has shown curcumin to have remarkable benefits for inflammation, viruses, protein handling, free radical damage, psoriasis, Crohn's disease, Alzheimer's, cystic fibrosis, Parkinson's, and more.

<u>Indole-3-Carbinol {I3C}, Lifelink</u> – A cruciferous vegetable extract that has anti cancer activity by regulating hormonal and cell signaling pathways. I3C sensitive cancers include those of the breast, prostrate, cervix, endometrium, colon, ovaries, lungs, white blood cells (leukemia) and skin. I3C has also shown

benefits with cervical dysplasia, herpes simplex virus, and Alzheimer's disease.

Super Cleanse, Irwin Naturals – Much more than just a simple cleansing formula with fibers, Super Cleanse includes botanicals traditionally used to nourish, stimulate and cleanse the colon and support the body's natural detoxification processes. Super Cleanse also provides probiotic support to enhance the process.

Milk Thistle Liver Cleanse, Irwin Naturals – Liver health is essential to the body's overall health, and Milk Thistle Liver Cleanse contains a proprietary blend of liver functioning and supporting ingredients. Botanicals in this product help to enhance vitality and promote healthy liver function.

Omega 3 (kids), Irwin Naturals – A gluten-free product that will nourish the brain and aid in concentration. Contains both DHA and EPA, both omega-3essential fatty acids and vitamin C, for anti-oxidant support.

Assist Dairy and Protein, Body Ecology – Designed to aid in the digestion ofproteins, including animal proteins, dairy foods, nuts, seeds, and legumes. This will help you get the most from what you eat by maximizing absorption and minimizing waste and toxicity.

Tachyonized Women's Ovarian Tonic, Tachyon – This organ-specific product nourishes and stimulates pituitary gland functions, particularly by acting as an ovary specific tonic addressing premenstrual stress and menopausalchanges. Contains chaste tree berry (vitex castus agnus)

Osteo Denx, Nikken – A revolutionary formula to help maintain strong and healthy bones. OsteoDenx is the only product with patented "syno-portin technology" that supports natural bone tissue growth. It literally helps rebuild bone density.

<u>Idebenone, Lifelink</u> – A COQ-10 variant, Idebenone works well in improving cognition, treating brain disorders, and protecting the body from low oxygen levels. Idebenone stimulates nerve growth factor (NGF) which also gives it the ability to be a neuroprotector and protect the mitochondria, which are the body's energy-producing cells.

<u>Acetyl-L-Carnitine, Lifelink</u> – Efficiently shuttles fat into the mitochondria for metabolic combustion and cellular energy. Acetyl-L-Carnitine also protects neurites in the brain. This combination, among other metabolic actions by Acetyl-L-Carnitine, gives it the ability to benefit many areas of wellness such as fibromyalgia, nerve injury, depression, Alzheimers, Parkinsons, and more.

<u>Carnosine, Lifelink</u> – Carnosine has potent anti-glycating effects. Glycation is a leading cause of age-related neurological, vascular, and eye problems. Nerve cells and muscle cells, when healthy contain high levels of carnosine, that keeps these cells young and healthy.

<u>Peelu, Starwest Botanicals</u> – Natural oral care to keep the mouth healthy and clean. Peelu products feature the gentle cleansing fibers and resins of the peelu tree (toothbrush tree), which have the ability to help whiten teeth, stimulate gums, remove plaque, and protect enamel from erosion.

DIETARY INTAKE SUGGESTIONS

The next pages will summarize our dietary intake program for optimal health, wellness, fitness, and performance.

The basic areas of concern within dietary intake include the following:

1} Determining your ideal/optimal health body weight and composition.

2} Determining your basal metabolism (resting/light activity) to support or attain this weight and body composition.

3} Dividing caloric intake properly among carbohydrate, protein, and fat.

To determine your body composition, you can visit any wellness center/clinic or purchase a scale that will record both weight and body composition.

IDEAL/OPTIMAL HEALTH WEIGHT AND BODY COMPOSITION

Name:_____ Date:_____

*Current Weight (lbs):____ X Current Body Fat Percent:____=
   Fat Weight (lbs)_____

*Current Weight (lbs):_____ — Fat Weight (lbs):_____ =
   Lean Body Weight. (lbs)_____

*Lean Weight (lbs)____ ÷ Ideal/Optimal Health Body Fat Percent____ =
   Ideal/Optimal Health Weight (lbs)_____

EXAMPLE

*Current Weight 247 lbs X Current Body Fat Percent 32% =
   Fat Weight: 79 lbs

*Current Weight 247 lbs - Fat Weight 79 lbs = Lean Body Weight 168 lbs

*Lean Body Weight 168 lbs ÷ Ideal/Optimal Health Body Fat Percent
   .15 (.85) = Ideal/Optimal Health Weight 197 lbs.

CLASSIFICATION	WOMEN	MEN
Essential Fat	11 – 14 percent	3 – 5 percent
Athletes	12 – 22 percent	5 – 13 percent
Fitness	16 – 25 percent	12 – 18 percent
Potential Risk	26 – 31 percent	19 – 24 percent
High Risk	32 percent plus	25 percent plus

DETERMINING BASAL METABOLISM

Basal Metabolism = calories/energy used
during rest and light daily activity

3.5 ml of oxygen per kg of body weight per minute

5 calories per liter of oxygen
(burn 5 calories for each liter of oxygen used)

Body weight in pounds ÷ 2.2 = body weight in kg

EXAMPLE

Weight in lbs = 225

225 ÷ 2.2 = 102 kg

102 kg X 3.5 = 357 ml oxygen per minute

357 ml oxygen per minute X 60 = 21,420 ml oxygen per hour

21,420 ml oxygen per hour X 24 = 514,080
ml oxygen per 24 hours

514,080 ml oxygen per 24 hours ÷ 1,000 = 514
liters of oxygen per 24 hours

514 liters oxygen X 5 = 2,570 calories (energy) per 24 hours

2,570 calories = basal metabolism

Always determine your basal metabolism based on your ideal/
optimal weight and body composition.

CALORIC BREAKDOWN

Caloric/Energy Expenditure Breakdown

*Basal Metabolism _____ calories/energy per 24-hour period
Energy used during rest and light daily activity – (see
determining basal metabolism sheet on page 40).

*Exercise/Activity:_____ calories/energy used
per exercise/activity session. See web site
www.healthstatus.com or www.healthfitcounter.com.

*Occupational:_____ calories/energy used per
day in occupation. See web site www.healthstatus.com
or www.healthfitcounter.com

*Specific Dynamic:_____ calories/energy used
consuming food – (figured in basal metabolism)

*Total Calories/Energy:_____ needed to meet your health,
wellness, fitness, and performance goals

These totals will assist you in achieving your ideal/optimal
health and goal body weight and body composition of
_____lbs and _____percent by supporting your
lean body weight (muscle, bones, organs, blood, ligaments,
etc.) and reducing adipose (fat) storage within and around
muscles, cells, and organs. This in turn will increase your
metabolism and support various health, wellness, fitness, and
performance parameters.

This total caloric/energy consumption will be achieved by
consuming 4 to 6 meals/snacks per day. Only water will be
consumed between each meal/snack.

This total caloric/energy consumption will be divided between the energy nutrients as follows:

*Carbohydrates:_____ grams:_____ calories
   (50 percent of total calories/energy)

*Protein:_____ grams:_____ calories
   (25 percent of total calories/energy)

*Fat:_____ grams:_____ calories –
   (25 percent of total calories/energy)

For carbohydrate and protein, divide calories by 4 to determine the number of grams. For fat, divide calories by 9.

For those with a goal of weight loss, the basal metabolism calories may suffice for total calories/energy needed. As your exercise/ activity level increases, you may need to add additional calories/ energy. Keep the added calories/energy in correct proportions of the energy nutrients – (carbohydrates, proteins, and fats).

For those with a goal of lean weight gain, you will need to add basal, exercise/activity, and occupational calories/energy. In addition, you still may need to add up to an additional 500 calories/energy. Again, keep added calories/energy in correct proportions of the energy nutrients (carbohydrates, proteins and fats).

For most individuals 50 percent carbohydrate and 25 percent protein and fat will be a good fit. Fast oxidizers may feel hungry with this breakdown and need to increase protein intake and reduce carbohydrate and fat intake. Slow oxidizers may feel full/bloated and need to increase complex/low glycemic carbohydrate intake and reduce protein and fat intake.

Fast Oxidizers: carbohydrate 40 percent, protein 40 percent, fat 20 percent

Slow Oxidizers: carbohydrate 60 percent, protein 20 percent, fat 20 percent

Unique Fitness Holistic Wellness Guideline Pyramid

Utilizing Nature's Innate Qualities & Universal Excellence

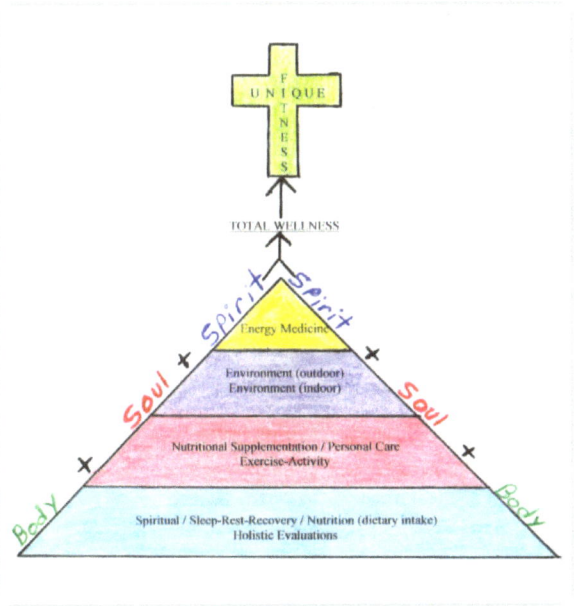

Implementing these will cause side effects: increased mood, energy, vitality, glowing skin, fitness, wisdom, financial

security, nurturing relationships, and more.
It's just something you will have to live with.

The following are excerpts from the Unique Fitness Holistic Wellness Guideline Pyramid and the coming book – *"The Unique Way To Wellness."*

*<u>Spiritual</u>:

You WERE NOT a mistake, for all your days are written in my book. (Psalm 139:15-16)

If you seek me with all your heart, you will find me. (Deuteronomy 4:29)

I am your FATHER, and I love you even as I love my SON, JESUS. (John 17:23)

*<u>Sleep/Rest/Recovery</u>:

Even mild sleep disruption in children can seriously interfere with cognitive development and learning ability.

70 million people in the United States have sleep disorders, – leading to slowed metabolism, increased fat storage, weight gain, lowered immunity, and more. (National Center on Sleep Disorders)

Financial losses in the United States due to sleep deprivation/ disorders total $100 billion per year due to-treatment, missed work, property damage, etc. (National Sleep Foundation)

*<u>Nutrition/Dietary Intake</u>:

75 percent of Americans are chronically dehydrated, which is the number 1 cause of daytime fatigue.

Protein consumption assists in the release of the hormones glucagon and cholecystakinin (CCK). Glucagon releases stored fat from adipose tissue to be used as an efficient energy source, while CCK sends satiety (fullness) messages to the brain to help prevent over-consumption.

When fruits and vegetables are picked or harvested un-ripened and shipped for several days, stored for several more days, and then sprayed with a gas to help ripen them overnight, they are almost completely void of all nutritional content because during the last days of ripening, these plants draw nutrients from the soil (if any nutrients are in the soil) to reach the full state of maturity.

*Holistic/Self Evaluations:

Thyroid temperature test: Take your temperature immediately in the morning before getting up or doing any activity. Leave thermometer in mouth for a full 3 minutes. Take readings five mornings in a row and average all readings after the fifth day. Females, if menstruating, begin readings four days after the start of the period.

> 97.8 to 98.2 degrees F: normal functioning thyroid

> Above 98.2 degrees F: hyperthyroid or possible infection

> Below 97.8 degrees F: possible hypothyroid

Muscle testing/applied kinesiology: A method to test supplements, foods, personal care products, etc with your personal energy field/flow, providing a virtual guarantee of product benefit.

Ice Cravings: May indicate an iron deficiency.

*Nutritional Supplementation:

The best health insurance you can invest in with an outstanding return on investment :- wellness.

Nature's answer to cost-preventive medicine. Can save billions in health care.

Foundational + Adaptogen + Targeted (for some) + Specialty (holistic medicine chest) = healthy cells→tissues→organs→systems = LIFE

*Exercise/Activity:

Two general types, including resistance/anaerobic and cardiovascular/aerobic. Depending on your wellness goals, incorporating one or both designed around the FITT principle will provide benefits. F= frequency, I = intensity, T = time, T = type.

If the benefits of exercise could be put in a pill, we would have the most powerful health-promoting medication available.

Brain scans of people over age fifty-five shows regular exercise helps significantly reduce loss of brain tissue (University of Illinois).

*Personal Care:

The skin is the largest organ in the body. What you put on your skin will absorb into your body and affect your health either positively or negatively.

Bad: Alcohol isopropyl (SD-40), diethonelamine (DEA), DMDM hydontoin and urea (imidazolidinyl), FD&C color pigments, fragrances, propylene glycol (PG), triclosan, are hormone disrupting and will slowly poison you.

Good: ASCIII, allantoin, algae extract, alpha hydroxy acids, liposomes, shea butter, sodium PCA, rosehip oil, etc.

*Outdoor Environment:

Japanese scientist have found that the same "safe" levels of fluoride commonly put into large segments of the U.S. water supply are capable of transmuting normal cells into cancer cells.

Chemtrails laid by military and commercial aircraft have us breathing ethylene dibromide, virally mutated molds, and nano-particles of aluminum, barium, and catonic polymer fibers, which are all detrimental to human and plant health.

Organic farming can help save the environment, largely due to conserving the precious topsoil. Many farming practices destroy up to 3 billion tons of topsoil every year which is a rate 7 times faster than mother nature can replenish it.

*Indoor Environment:

Poor indoor air ranks among the top 5 environmental risks to public health. (American Lung Association and 3M)

Feng shui utilizes natural elements and the art of placement to bring equilibrium and harmony to your environment.

Electromagnetic fields (EMF's) can cause changes in living cells that are detrimental to human health, resulting in cancers, miscarriages, childhood leukemia, and more. Protect yourself with tachyonized zero-point energy products.

*Energy Medicine:

The human body has an electrical frequency, and much about a person's health can be determined by it.

Every disease has a frequency. Certain frequencies can prevent the development of disease, while others will destroy disease.

Magnetic energy is natural earth energy that is essential to the life of every cell. Far-infrared energy is the wave length of life. Negative ions are nature's life-enhancing particles. Tachyon energy is zero point energy for body/soul/spirit.

RESOURCES

The following web addresses will provide invaluable
   information addressing each phase of the Unique Fitness
   Holistic Wellness Guideline Pyramid.

ULTRA LABORATORIES = www.ultralaboratories.com
   The additive-free company. Nutritional supplements,
   personal care products, fruitrients super foods.

IRWIN NATURALS = www.irwinnaturals.com
   Are you serious about potency? Nutritional supplements,
   children's supplements, great cleansing products.

STARWEST BOTANICLAS = www.starwest-botanicals.com
   Innovative leader in superior quality botanical products.
   Wide variety of natural wellness products.

GRAINFIELDS AUSTRALIA = www.grainfieldsaustralia.com
   Ferm flora, a natural organic fermentation process. Nature's
   food fermented for vibrant health.

LIFELINK = www.lifelinknet.com
   Nutraceuticals and nootropics for anti-aging. Because good
   health is not an accident.

OMEGA NUTRITION = www.omeganutrition.com
   The original flaxseed oil company. Certified organic
   omegaflo oils, the power of essential fatty acids.

NATURE'S GATE = www.naturesgatebeauty.com
   Personal care at its best. Hair, bath, skin, deodorant,

oral, facial, acne, and sun care, all from certified natural botanicals.

BEEHIVE BOTANICALS = www.beehivebotanicals.com
Purity, integrity, and quality since 1972. Royal jelly, bee pollen, bee propolis, body and bath.

HEMP OIL OF CANADA = www.hempoilcan.com
The seed you need. Hemp seed oil contains omega-6, omega-3, GLA, and 75 percent – 80 percent polyunsaturated fatty acids, the highest in the plant kingdom and unique among seed oils.

BODY ECOLOGY = www.bodyecology.com
Recovering your health and rebuilding your immunity. Fermented probiotic foods for a healthy inner ecosystem.

CLAYTON NATURALS = www.claytonnaturals.com
All vegetarian, cruelty-free ingredients with 100 percent ethnically -crafted and/or organic herb formulas.

BIONEERS = www.bioneers.org
Breakthrough solutions for people and planet. Inspiring a shift to live on earth in ways that honor the web of life, each other, and future generations.

NIKKEN = www.mynikken.com
The wellness home company. Bringing wellness home for more than thirty years. Discover it, live it.

TACHYON = www.planet-tachyon.com/kyle
Advanced Tachyon Technologies, Inc. gives us a new paradigm in holistic health. Tachyon is the source of all frequencies for healthy body/soul/spirit.

ALACER CORP = www.emergenc.com
Little packets of kapow. Over twenty varieties of vitamin drink mixes that will jump start your wellness.

DR. BRONNER'S MAGIC SOAPS = www.bronner.com
Dr. Bronner's magic soaps are synonymous with old world quality and time-honored simplicity. No synthetic junk.

DAVINCI LABORATORIES = www.davincilabs.com
For over thirty-nine years, DaVinci Labs has developed leading edge–high-quality formulations for both human and animal needs.

NATURAL PRODUCTS ASSOCIATION = www. naturalproductsassoc.org
Promoting natural products for healthy lifestyles and improving quality of life for consumers worldwide.

ORGANIC CONSUMERS ASSOCIATION = www. organicconsumers.org
Campaigning for health, justice, sustainability, peace, and democracy For socially responsible consumers.

WESTON A PRICE FOUNDATIONS = www.westonaprice.org
For wise traditions in food, farming, and the healing arts through education, research, and activism.

AMERICAN NATUROPATHIC MEDICAL ASSOC. = www. anma.com
The nations oldest and largest American association of naturopathic physicians. Exploring new frontiers of mind, body, medicine, and health. "Doctor do no harm."

AMERICAN HERBALIST GUILD = www. americanherbalistguild.com
Honoring diversity in herbal medicine, ranging from traditional indigenous models of herbalism to modern clinical phytotherapy.

COALITION OF NATURAL HEALTH = www.naturalhealth.org
National organization promoting natural health freedom and protecting the rights of natural health practitioners.

NATIONAL HEALTH FEDERATION = www.thenhf.com
The NHF is a consumer education health freedom organization working to protect individual rights to choose and consume healthy food, take supplements, and use alternative therapies without government restrictions.

VEGETARIAN RESOURCE GROUP = www.vrg.org
Dedicated to educating the public on vegetarianism and the interrelated issues of healthy nutrition, ecology, ethics, and world hunger.

NUTRITIONAL HEALTH ALLIANCE = www.nha2004.com
Protecting your rights. The NHA is one of the most active political organizations in the nutritional health community.

TRINITY BROADCASTING NETWORK = www.tbn.org
America's most watched faith channel featuring a wide variety of inspirational programming for all ages.

AMERICAN CENTER FOR LAW AND JUSTICE = www.aclj.com
Dedicated to the ideal that religious freedom and freedom of speech are inalienable, God given rights.

BOTT RADIO = www.bottradionetwork.com
Getting the word of God into the people of God through integrity, service, strength, and quality.

KLTT RADIO = www.670kltt.com
Colorado's Christian station – (670 AM radio). Read, listen, learn, grow, get the real news.

KJLT RADIO = www.kjlt.org
GOD created us for his glory. Our reason for being here is to glorify Him. Bible search, daily devotionals, Bible challenge.

ABOUT THE AUTHOR

Kyle believes that life and wellness are journeys, not destinations. The Unique Fitness Holistic Wellness Guideline Pyramid is merely a continuation of this journey. This journey began early in life through grade school, junior high, high school, and college athletics, which set the stage for a lifetime of interest within the disciplines of health, wellness, fitness, and performance.

Kyle firmly believes that you have to practice what you preach while becoming a living role model to earn the respect and trust of everyone seeking to join in on the journey. Kyle does this by following the Unique Fitness Holistic Wellness Guideline Pyramid.

Kyle has developed an unshakeable desire, belief, and passion to continue this wellness journey and has many years (more than thirty) of formal and informal education within such diverse disciplines as exercise science/ wellness, holistic nutrition, herbology, subtle energy wellness, bodywork, traditional naturopathy, athletic training, teacher education, iridology, applied kinesiology, therapeutic nutrition, spirituality/Christianity, and more. The Unique Fitness Holistic Wellness Guideline Pyramid and programs were developed from this education.

Clayton College of Natural Health. Master of Science in Holistic Nutrition, March 2011

Nikken, Inc., Humans Being More Self Actualization Training and Certification, April 1997 & 1998

International Correspondence Schools, Fitness and Nutrition Certification, April 1994

Sports Telesis, Inc., Individual Nutrition and Fitness Technology Certification, August 1994

Great Plains Regional Medical Center, Exercise Science and Wellness Internship, June 1993

Wayne State College, Bachelor of Science in Exercise Science and Wellness - Athletic Training, May 1992

National Association for Sport and Physical Education, Outstanding Physical Education Major, May 1991

Wayne State College, Bachelor of Arts in K-12 Health and Physical Education-Coaching Endorsement, May 1991

Kyle worked as a certified nutrition and fitness consultant for Gold's Gym Aerobic and Fitness Center before developing the Unique Fitness Holistic Wellness Guideline Pyramid. Since early 1994 he has pursued the potential of the human body/soul/spirit to be well through UNIQUE ways→ Utilizing Nature's Innate Qualities & Universal Excellence.

Kyle also firmly believes in continually educating oneself and staying current with the latest developments in the health, wellness, fitness, and performance disciplines. Advanced Tachyon Technologies, Inc. and The Kingdom College of Natural Health provide this cutting-edge education.

Kyle McCormick, M.S., I.N.F.T.C. {Sportelesis. Inc.}

Unique Fitness
Ogallala, NE. 69153
uniquefitness1@yahoo.com
(308) 289-5806
www.uniqftns.com (coming soon)

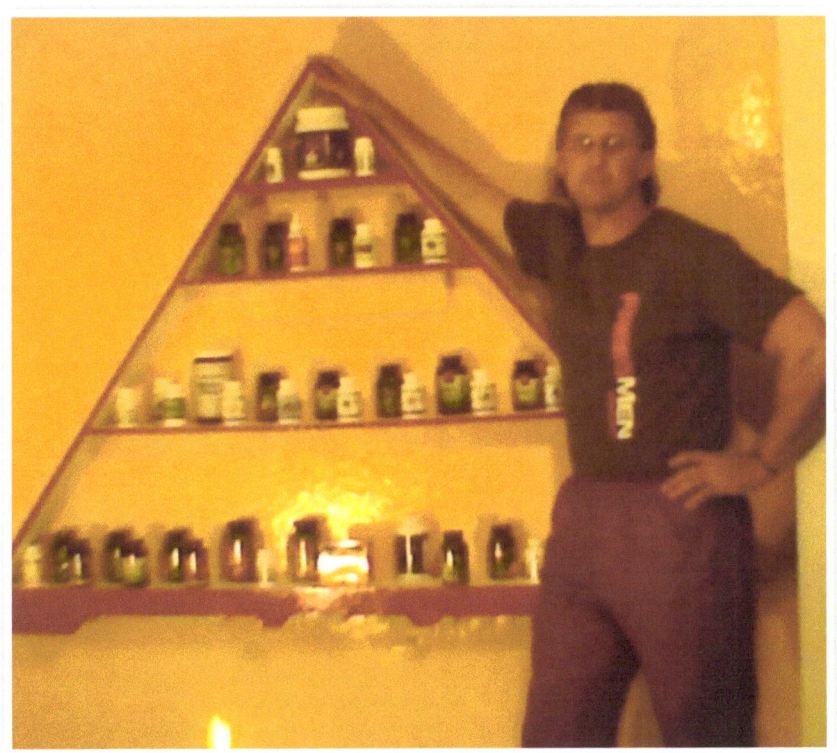

REFERENCES

"Ask Dr. Zarkov," Lifelink: Nutraceuticals and Nootropics for Anti-Aging, accessed December 21, 2009.

www.lifelinknet.com/siteresources/askdrzarkov/2009/08/ vitaminD-flu.asp Balch, J., M.D., and Balch, P., C.N.C. *Prescription for Nutritional Healing.* Garden City Park: Avery Publishing Group, 1997.

Boyle, M. M.S., R.D. and Whitney E., PhD., R.D. *Personal Nutrition.* St. Paul West Publishing Company, 1989.

"Breakthrough in Understanding Anti-Cancer Effect of Vitamin C." Retrieved December 21, 2009 from www.lifelinknet. com/siteresources/suppsinthenews/2005/01/vitamin-c-anticancer.asp.

Cichoke, A., D.C., M.A. *Enzymes & Enzyme Therapy: How To Jump-Start Your Way To Lifelong Good Health.* Los Angeles: Keats Publishing, 2000.

Colgan, M. PhD., C.C.N. *Optimum Sports Nutrition.* Ronkonkoma, NY: Advanced Research Press, 1993.

Cousens, G., M.D. "Super Rejuvenation Food For The Brain." Retrieved March 5, 2010 from www.planet-tachyon.com/kyle

Gaemi, S., ED.D., R.D. *Eating Wisely For Hormonal Health.* Oakland, CA. New Harbinger Publications, 2004.

Gerber, R., M.D. *Vibrational Medicine.* Rochester, VT. Bear and Company, 2001.

Gittleman, A., M.S., C.N.S. *The Fat Flush Plan.* New York: McGraw-Hill, 2002.

Hashimoto, A. "Mineral Chelates, Salts and Colloids." Retrieved March 19, 2010 from www.delano.com/articles/mineral-formscompound.html.

Khalsa, D., M.D. *Food As Medicine, How To Use Diet, Vitamins, Juices and Herbs for a Healthier and Longer Life.* New York: Atria Books, 2003.

LifeLink. "Athletes, Autism, ADHD: The Magnesium Connection." Lifelink, Inc., 2007.

LifeLink. "Osteoporosis and Cancer Have Worn Out Their Welcome. Let's Give Them the Boot!" Lifelink, Inc., 2007.

Margen, S., M.D. *The Wellness Encyclopedia of Food and Nutrition.* New York: Rebus, 1992.

Mindell, E., R.P.h., PhD, with Mundis, H. *Earl Mindell's New Vitamin Bible.* New York: Warner Books, 2009.

Null, G., PhD. *Power Aging: The Revolutionary Program to Control the Symptoms of Aging Naturally.* Stamford, CT. Penguin Group, Inc., 2003.

Stengler, M., N.D. *The Natural Physicians Healing Therapies: Proven Remedies That Medical Doctors Don't Know About.* Stamford, CT. Prentice Hall Press, 2001.

Stine, J. "Lactoferrin: The First Food for Life." Retrieved February 26, 2006 from www.ehot.com/smartbasics/1_lactoferrin.html.

"Let food be your medicine and medicine be your food. Who so ever gives these things no consideration and is ignorant of them, how can he understand the diseases of man?"
Hippocrates, ca. 400 BC

"No physician can ever say that any disease is incurable. To say so blasphemes God, blasphemes nature, and depreciates the great architect of creation. The disease does not exist, regardless of how terrible it may be, for which God has not provided the corresponding cure."
Paracelsus, – The Father of Pharmacology

"All that mankind needs for good health and healing is provided in nature. The challenge to science is to find it."
Paracelsus, – The Father of Pharmacology

"In the arts of life man invents nothing, but in the arts of death he outdoes nature herself and produces by chemistry and machinery all the slaughter of plague, pestilence and famine."
George Bernard Shaw

Money Savings: Over a five year period, appropriate use of dietary supplements would improve the health of countless individuals and save the nation more than $24 billion in health care costs. The individual savings would be staggering: at least $1700 per year for every man, woman and child in the United States.
Dietary Supplement Education Alliance (DSEA)

www.ingramcontent.com/pod-product-compliance
Lightning Source LLC
Chambersburg PA
CBHW050811290526

45792CB00001B/67